The UTI Handbook

Your Guide to Urinary Tract Infection Symptoms and Solutions

Harmony Royce

DEDICATION

This book is dedicated to the innumerable people who are looking for answers, respite, and long-term remedies, as well as to those who have felt the pain and frustration of urinary tract infections. I hope it gives you the information, insight, and optimism you need to take charge of your health and live a life free from UTIs.

I would like to express my gratitude to my family, friends, and medical professionals for their constant support and dedication to this effort.

DISCLAIMER

The UTI Handbook: Your Guide to Urinary Tract Infection Symptoms and Solutions contains information that is meant primarily for educational purposes and should not be used in place of expert medical advice, diagnosis, or treatment. If you have any questions about a medical condition or treatment, you should always consult your doctor or another trained healthcare professional.

Any negative effects or repercussions arising from the usage of any information in this book are not the responsibility of the author or publisher. For the proper advice and treatment, please see a healthcare provider if you are exhibiting signs of a urinary tract infection or any other health issues.

CONTENTS

ACKNOWLEDGMENTS

I would like to express my sincere appreciation to everyone who helped create *The UTI Handbook.*

Above all, I want to express my sincere gratitude to my family and friends for their constant encouragement, tolerance, and support along this journey. Your confidence in me inspired and encouraged me to finish this job.

A special thank you to the scholars, medical specialists, and healthcare practitioners whose knowledge influenced this book's content. Your priceless advice and commitment to enhancing patient care have helped me deliver accurate and trustworthy information.

I also like to thank the design team, editors, and proofreaders that made this book possible. Your meticulousness and dedication to quality made this work both educational and readable.

Last but not least, I dedicate my book to the innumerable people who suffer from UTIs. I hope this guide gives you the information and tools you need to better understand your health, get relief, and live a life free from UTI discomfort.

We appreciate your support and donations, everyone.

CHAPTER 1

UNDERSTANDING URINARY TRACT INFECTIONS (UTIs)

Every year, millions of people worldwide suffer from urinary tract infections (UTIs), one of the most prevalent medical disorders. This chapter examines the basic elements of UTIs, including a thorough grasp of their terminology, the urinary system's structure, and the various infection kinds.

1.1 An Overview and Definition of UTIs

Any infection that affects any of the kidneys, ureters, bladder, or urethra is referred to as a urinary tract infection (UTI). Although fungi and viruses can occasionally be the source of certain diseases, bacteria are the main culprits.

Important Features:

- Common Culprits: Escherichia coli, or E. coli, is the cause of 80–90% of simple UTIs, which frequently start in the gastrointestinal tract.

- Because of the shorter length of the female urethra, which makes it easier for germs to enter the bladder, women are more likely to get UTIs than males.

- Some people have recurrent UTIs, which are characterized by three or more infections in a year or two infections in a six-month period.

Signs and symptoms:

Decreased UTI (Urethra and Bladder):

- A burning feeling when urinating.

- Urinating frequently and urgently, even when the bladder is not full.

- Urine that is hazy, pungent, or has blood in it.

- A slight soreness in the pelvis.

Kidneys Upper UTI:

- Fatigue, chills, and fever.

- Vomiting or feeling sick.

- Pain near the ribs in the side or upper back.

The Importance of Knowing About UTIs

- **Health Impact:** If left untreated, UTIs can cause

serious side effects as sepsis or kidney infections (pyelonephritis).

- **Economic Burden:** Because UTIs necessitate frequent medical visits, diagnostic testing, and treatments, they lead to substantial healthcare expenses.

Understanding the urinary tract's structure and the many kinds of infections can help us better understand how these diseases develop and how to treat them.

1.2 The Urinary Tract's Anatomy: Important Structures

Knowing the anatomy of the urinary tract is crucial to understanding how UTIs arise and impact the body. Each of the four major structures that make up the urinary system is essential to the production, storage, and excretion of urine.

Important Elements:

1. Kidneys:

- Below the rib cage, on either side of the spine, are bean-shaped organs.

- Its function is to filter the blood of waste materials, poisons, and extra fluid.

- Control the synthesis of red blood cells, blood pressure, and electrolytes.

Relation to UTIs:

- If left untreated, upper urinary tract infections (UTIs) can cause kidney damage.

2. Ureters:

- The narrow tubes that carry urine from the kidneys to the bladder are known as ureters.

- Its function is to guarantee a one-way urine flow by using peristaltic movements.

Relation to UTIs: Urinary blockages or reflux can make people more vulnerable to infections.

3. Bladder

- The bladder is a muscular, hollow organ situated in the pelvic.

- Its purpose is to temporarily hold pee until it is expelled.

Relation to UTIs: Bacteria frequently settle here, resulting in bladder infections, or cystitis.

4. Urethra

- The urethra is a tube that transports urine from the bladder to the outside of the body.
- Its function is to act as the urine's departure point.

Relation to UTIs: In females, its closeness to the anus enhances exposure to microorganisms.

Urinary Tract Protective Mechanisms:

- **Urine Flow:** Frequent urination aids in the removal of germs.
- **Mucosal Barriers:** The lining of the urinary tract prevents bacteria from adhering.
- **Immune Responses:** Urinary tract infections are actively fought by the body.

The significance of preserving urinary tract health is highlighted by the fact that infections can result from disruptions in these defense mechanisms.

1.3 Urinary Tract Infection Types: Upper vs. Lower

Depending on where they occur in the urinary system, UTIs can be broadly classified. Because upper and lower tract infections range greatly in severity and consequences, this distinction is essential for diagnosis and therapy.

Lower UTIs:

- Affected Areas: Urinary tract and bladder.

Common Conditions:

- **Cystitis:** Bladder inflammation.

- Inflammation of the urethra is known as urethritis.

Symptoms:

- Burning feeling when urinating.

- Urinating frequently.

- Lower abdominal pain or pressure.

Causes:

- poor hygiene.

- Sexual activities.

- The use of certain contraceptives, such as spermicides or diaphragms.

Upper urinary tract infections:

- **Affected Areas:** Urinary tract and kidneys.

Common Conditions:

- **Pyelonephritis:** Kidney inflammation.

Symptoms:

- Chills and fever.

- The back hurts close to the kidneys.

- Vomiting and nausea.

Causes:

- Lower urinary tract infections that progress to the kidneys without treatment.

- Anatomical anomalies or obstructions in the urinary tract.

Key Differences:

Feature	Lower UTI	Upper UTI
Severity	Mild to moderate	Potentially life-threatening
Primary Symptoms	Localized discomfort	Systemic symptoms (fever, chills)

Treatment	Oral antibiotics	Intravenous antibiotics (in severe cases)

Complications to Keep an Eye on:

- **Recurrent Infections:** Usually arise from insufficient bacterial elimination.
- Long-term infections can cause scarring and decreased kidney function.
- A serious, sometimes fatal reaction to an infection is sepsis.

In order to manage upper and lower UTIs, guarantee a full recovery, and minimize the risk of complications, a proper diagnosis and focused therapy are essential.

Readers who have a basic awareness of UTIs, their anatomical context, and their classifications will be better able to identify symptoms, realize the value of prompt treatment, and take preventative action.

CHAPTER 2

UTI Causes and Risk Factors

Effective prevention and treatment of urinary tract infections (UTIs) depend on knowledge of their causes and risk factors. This chapter examines the medical, lifestyle, and biological factors that contribute to the development of UTIs, highlighting how these factors interact to increase susceptibility.

2.1 E. coli and Other Common Bacterial Causes

Escherichia coli (E. coli) is the main bacterium responsible for the great majority of UTIs. In addition to highlighting additional bacteria that cause infections, this section explores the microbiology of UTIs.

The most prevalent cause is E. coli, a bacterium that is frequently present in the gastrointestinal (GI) tract. Although it is usually innocuous in the gastrointestinal tract, infections may result from its presence in the urinary tract.

The mechanism of infection is as follows:

E. coli adheres to the urinary tract's epithelial lining by use of specialized structures known as fimbriae. The bacteria grow and create biofilms once they are attached, shielding them from antibiotics and immunological reactions.

Additional Bacterial Infections

While 80–90% of simple UTIs are caused by E. coli, other bacteria can also cause infections, such as:

- The bacteria Klebsiella pneumoniae is frequently found in hospital-acquired UTIs.
- Linked to antibiotic resistance and catheter use.

Proteus mirabilis:

- Generates urease, an enzyme that raises the alkalinity of urine and encourages the development of stones.
- This is frequently observed in complex UTIs.
- One of the main causes of UTIs in young women who engage in sexual activity is Staphylococcus saprophyticus.

In comparison to other pathogens, it causes infections that are milder.

- The bacteria Enterococcus faecalis is frequently found in elderly patients or individuals who have had extended hospital admissions.
- It may result in infections that are resistant to antibiotics.

Causes by Viral and Fungal Agents

- **Candida Species:** Fungal UTIs are uncommon and usually affect people with urinary catheters or those with weakened immune systems.
- Adenoviruses: Although they are rare, viral UTIs can result in hemorrhagic cystitis, especially in children and those with compromised immune systems.

To choose the best course of action and avoid recurring infections, it is essential to identify the precise organism causing the infection.

2.2 Risk Factors Associated with Lifestyle and Hygiene

Although bacterial infections cause UTIs, specific lifestyle decisions and personal hygiene habits can foster an infection-friendly environment. The chance of getting a UTI can be considerably decreased by taking care of these things.

Hygiene Practices:

Incorrect Wiping Method:

- Wiping from the back to the front increases the risk of infection by transferring bacteria from the anal area to the urethra.
- The answer is to teach people how to wipe properly, especially young females.

Inadequate Perineal Hygiene:

- Bacteria can flourish close to the urethral opening due to poor genital hygiene.
- Maintaining a balanced microbiota can be facilitated by routinely washing with mild, unscented soap.

Intercourse:

Bacterial Transfer:

- Intercourse has the potential to transmit bacteria into the urinary tract.

- Women are at greater risk because of their shorter urethras.

Preventive Measures:

- To eliminate microorganisms, urinate both before and after sexual activity.
- Water-based lubricants are used to avoid microtrauma and discomfort.

Clothes Options:

tight pants or underwear:

- Limits ventilation and produces a damp atmosphere, which encourages the growth of microorganisms.
- It is advised to wear cotton underwear for improved breathability.

Hydration and Urination Practices:

Low Fluid Intake:

- Consuming too little water limits the normal flushing mechanism of the urinary system by reducing urine production.

Postponing Urination:

- Prolonged holding of urine gives bacteria more time to grow.

People can greatly reduce their chances of getting UTIs by changing to a healthier lifestyle and practicing better cleanliness.

2.3 Health Issues That Raise the Risk of UTIs

By compromising the urinary tract's natural defenses or fostering conditions that encourage the growth of germs, several medical disorders make people more susceptible to UTIs.

Abnormalities in Structure

Urinary Tract Obstructions:

- Disorders such as kidney stones or tumors can block the flow of urine, which gives germs a place to grow.
- Vesicoureteral reflux (VUR) is a congenital disease that increases the risk of kidney infections by causing urine to flow backward from the bladder to the kidneys.

Long-Term Medical Conditions

Diabetes Mellitus:

- Bacterial growth may be encouraged by elevated

blood sugar levels.

- Diabetics' weakened immune systems make them even more vulnerable.

Chronic Kidney Disease (CKD):

- Decreases the kidneys' capacity to eliminate pathogens and waste.

Neurological Conditions

Neurogenic Bladder:

- Conditions like multiple sclerosis or spinal cord injuries can interfere with the bladder's natural ability to empty, which can result in partial emptying and frequent urinary tract infections.

Hormonal Changes

Pregnancy:

- Hormonal shifts and uterine pressure on the bladder might restrict urine flow, raising infection risk.

- The vaginal and urethral linings may become thinner due to decreased estrogen levels, which will lessen their capacity to fend against bacterial colonization.

Medical Equipment and Procedures

When urinary catheters are used for an extended period of time, bacteria are directly introduced into the urinary system.

Surgical Interventions:

- Patients having urological procedures may develop postoperative infections.

Weakened Immune System: People with weakened immune systems, such as those receiving chemotherapy or having HIV/AIDS, are more susceptible to urinary tract infections.

The complexity of UTIs is highlighted by this thorough examination of their etiology and risk factors. Understanding these elements can help create focused preventative plans, lower the risk of infections, and guarantee improved urinary health.

CHAPTER 3

Common UTI Symptoms

Early detection and efficient treatment of a urinary tract infection (UTI) depend on the ability to recognize its common symptoms. UTIs, which are brought on by bacterial invasion of the urinary system, have unique, frequently bothersome symptoms that can greatly affect day-to-day functioning. This chapter explores the main symptoms, including their underlying causes and potential health consequences.

3.1 An explanation of painful urination (dysuria)

One of the main signs of a urinary tract infection is painful urination, or dysuria. It describes pain, scorching, or stinging feelings that come with urinating.

Causes of dysuria in UTIs
- The lining of the urethra becomes irritated by

17

bacterial infections, which makes it sensitive and unpleasant to pass urine. This is one of the causes of dysuria in UTIs.

- The lower abdomen may experience pain when the bladder wall becomes inflamed, which can be made worse by urinating. This condition is known as bladder inflammation (cystitis).

- **Urine Acidity:** Infected urine frequently becomes more acidic, which exacerbates the irritation of tissues that are already inflamed.

Characteristics of Dysuria

- The burning sensation is a common description of dysuria, which is caused by inflamed tissues along the urinary system.

- Women may experience pain in the vicinity of the urethral opening.

- Men frequently complain about penile pain.

- **Severity**: Depending on how severe the infection is, the pain can be anything from slight discomfort to a strong, stinging agony.

Differential Diagnosis

- Although dysuria is a typical symptom of a urinary tract infection, it can also be a sign of other illnesses such as vaginal infections (e.g., bacterial vaginosis or yeast infections).
- Sexually transmitted infections, such as gonorrhea or chlamydia.
- Sexual activities can cause urethral damage or discomfort.

In order to differentiate UTIs from other causes of painful urination, early medical assessment is crucial.

3.2 Strong and Regular Urinary Urges

An increased frequency and desire to urinate, which frequently interferes with sleep and everyday routines, is another hallmark symptom of UTIs.

Why Do These Symptoms Occur?

Bladder wall inflammation is caused by irritation of bladder receptors, which gives the brain continual messages that the bladder is full.

Decreased Bladder Capacity:

- Infections can cause the bladder to become too sensitive, which reduces its capacity to comfortably store pee.
- **Incomplete Emptying:** Inflammation and bacteria can hinder the bladder's capacity to empty completely, resulting in frequent urination.

Features of Urgency and Frequency

Persistent want to Urinate:

- People frequently have an unrelieved want to urinate again, even right after voiding.

little pee Volumes:

- Despite the urgent feeling, urination may only result in little volumes of pee.
- The need to urinate frequently at night, which interferes with sleep patterns, is known as nocturia.

Social and Psychological Effects

Stress and Anxiety:

- An ongoing sense of urgency can lead to anxiety and make it hard to concentrate on duties.

Quality of Life:

- Travel, social interactions, and employment may be

hampered by frequent restroom breaks.

Early management and enough hydration can help lessen these symptoms and lower the chance of consequences.

3.3 Discolored, hazy, or foul-smelling urine

Urine changes in color, odor, and appearance are frequently signs of a UTI. White blood cells, bacteria, and other inflammatory byproducts in the urinary system cause these symptoms.

Cloudy Urine

Pus and White Blood Cells (Pyuria):

- White blood cells are released into the urine as a result of the immune system's reaction to bacterial invasion, which causes the urine to appear cloudy.

Mucus and Cellular Debris:

- Dead bacteria and sloughed-off cells can further contaminate the urine as the condition worsens.

Urine With an Odor

Bacterial Metabolism:

- Ammonia and other waste products are produced by bacteria such as *E. coli* and give off a pungent, disagreeable smell.

Infection Severity:

- The degree of the infection is frequently correlated with the strength of the odor.

Discolored Urine:

Hematuria (Blood in Urine):

- Inflammation from a UTI can result in mild bleeding, which can make the urine pink, red, or brown.

- Severe infections are more likely to cause visible hematuria.

- Dehydration, which is prevalent during UTIs, can concentrate urine and enhance its color, resulting in dark yellow or tea-colored urine.

Important Factors in Diagnosis

Urine characteristic changes are not unique to UTIs and can coexist with other illnesses like:

- Kidney stones, which cause blood and hazy urine.

- Dehydration, as seen by black urine

- Some drugs or foods (such rifampin or beets) that change the look of urine.

Knowing When to Get Medical Help

- Constant alterations in the look or smell of urine.
- Fever and chills are examples of accompanying systemic symptoms that could point to a more serious infection.

People can identify the early warning signs and seek timely medical assistance by being aware of the common symptoms of a UTI. In addition to guaranteeing successful treatment, early detection lowers the chance of side effects including kidney infections or recurring episodes.

CHAPTER 4

Lower UTI (Cystitis) Symptoms

Cystitis, another name for lower urinary tract infections (UTIs), mostly affects the bladder and urethra. Even though cystitis symptoms are restricted to the lower urinary system, they can nevertheless be quite upsetting and uncomfortable. It is crucial to identify these signs early in order to avoid consequences and guarantee timely treatment. The most typical signs of lower urinary tract infections, their underlying causes, and their effects on health are examined in this chapter.

4.1 Bladder or Pelvic Area Pain

One of the hallmarks of cystitis is pain that is restricted to the bladder or pelvis. From a slight aching to severe pressure or cramping, this discomfort might vary widely.

Features of Pelvic or Bladder Pain:

Sensation and Location:

- Pain is frequently experienced above the pubic bone in the lower abdomen. It could show up as a heaviness, intense pain, or dull soreness.

Worsening Pain During Urination:

- The inflammatory tissues may produce increased discomfort as the bladder contracts to release urine.
- Radiating discomfort can cause pain to radiate to other regions, such the groin or lower back.

Root produces of discomfort

Bladder Wall Inflammation:

- An infection leads to swelling of the bladder lining, which produces discomfort and irritation.

Pressure from Urine Retention:

- Cystitis patients frequently experience incomplete bladder emptying, which makes pressure and discomfort worse.

Muscle Spasms:

- Inflammation may cause the detrusor muscle, which contracts involuntarily, causing the pain to worsen.

Distinguishing This Condition from Others

It is not only cystitis that causes pelvic or bladder pain. Similar symptoms can also be caused by the following conditions:

- **Interstitial Cystitis:** Prolonged inflammation of the bladder that is not caused by a bacterial infection.
- Muscle strains or spasms in the pelvic area are indicative of pelvic floor dysfunction.
- Endometriosis and pelvic inflammatory disease are examples of gynecological disorders.

In order to address the root problem and offer relief, prompt evaluation and diagnosis are essential.

4.2 Fatigue with Low-Grade Fever

Although they are less common than upper urinary tract infections, modest systemic symptoms like weariness and a low-grade fever can occasionally happen with lower UTIs.

Low-Grade Fever:

The following are the features of fever in cystitis:

- The usual temperature range is 37.5°C to 38°C (99.5°F to 100.4°F).

- Chills may accompany the illness, but unless the infection has spread, a significant fever is rare.

Fever Mechanism in UTIs:

- Pyrogens, which cause an increase in body temperature, are released by the immune system in response to bacterial invasion.
- Fever of low grade indicates a localized infection with little to no systemic involvement.

Malaise and Fatigue

Impact of Inflammation:

- Lethargy and fatigue can be caused by immunological activation and inflammatory processes.

Sleep Disruption:

- Symptoms like frequent urination or soreness in the bladder can cause sleep disturbances, which exacerbates exhaustion.

Energy Expenditure:

- People feel exhausted after fighting an infection since it takes metabolic energy.

When to Worry: Treatment for cystitis should alleviate fever and tiredness. Nonetheless, the following symptoms call for medical intervention:

- A fever that is higher than 38°C (100.4°F).

- Fatigue that doesn't go away or gets worse even after drinking enough water and getting enough sleep.

- Side effects including nausea or flank discomfort could be signs that a kidney infection is developing.

4.3 Hematuria, or mild blood in the urine

Blood in the urine, or hematuria, can vary in intensity and is a potential sign of cystitis. It can give the urine a pink, crimson, or brown tinge and manifest as visible blood or microscopic blood that can only be detected by laboratory testing.

Features of Hematuria in Cystitis
Microscopic Hematuria:

- Usually detected by urine testing, this condition is common in cystitis.

- Visible (Gross) Hematuria: This is uncommon in lower urinary tract infections, but when it does occur, it can result in an obvious urine discoloration.

Inflamed Blood Vessels:

- Bacterial infection destroys the bladder lining, exposing small blood vessels and causing mild bleeding. This is one of the causes of hematuria in cystitis.

Increased Bladder Pressure:

- Inflammation-induced discomfort and frequent urination might worsen vascular damage.

Distinguishing Other Causes of Hematuria

Although hematuria is linked to cystitis, it can also be caused by other illnesses like:

- Kidney stones can cause damage to the lining of the urinary tract due to their sharp crystals.
- One of the main warning signs for bladder cancer is persistent, painless hematuria.
- **Trauma:** Damage to the urinary tract resulting from intense exercise or catheterization.

Clinical Importance

When cystitis is treated with the right antibiotics, mild

hematuria usually goes away. Further testing, such as imaging or cystoscopy, is necessary to rule out serious underlying diseases in cases with persistent or recurring hematuria.

People can more easily identify lower urinary tract infections (UTIs) and seek prompt treatment if they are aware of their symptoms. Early treatment of these symptoms can minimize discomfort and lower the chance that they will develop into more serious infections.

CHAPTER 5

Upper UTI (Kidney Infection) Symptoms

Upper urinary tract infections, sometimes referred to as kidney infections or pyelonephritis, are a more serious type of UTI that, if untreated, can cause serious problems. Kidney infections impact the kidneys, which are essential organs in charge of filtering blood and creating urine, in contrast to lower UTIs, which are mainly restricted to the bladder and urethra. Upper urinary tract infections have more severe, systemic symptoms that need to be treated right away. The main symptoms of upper urinary tract infections are thoroughly examined in this chapter, with a focus on their etiology, clinical importance, and treatment implications.

5.1 Sweating, chills, and a high fever

A high temperature, frequently accompanied by chills and excessive perspiration, is one of the telltale symptoms of an upper urinary tract infection. These signs show that the infection has moved beyond the lower urinary tract and point to a systemic reaction to the illness.

Features of Fever in Kidney Infections

Severity and Temperature:

- A severe fever usually reaches 38°C (100.4°F) or higher, and its maximum temperature can reach 39.5°C (103°F).

- The fever is frequently sporadic, accompanied by excessive sweating as the body tries to control its temperature.

- Uncontrollable chills or shivering episodes are frequent and happen as the body responds to bacterial toxins.

- Sweating fits usually follow chills, which causes a large loss of fluid.

Night Sweats:

- Sweating can happen at night, soaking bed linens and necessitating comfort and hydration.

Fundamental Processes

Immune Activation:

- The body increases its temperature to make the environment less conducive to the growth of bacteria.

- The hypothalamus raises body temperature in response to pyrogens, which are chemicals secreted by immune cells.

- **Systemic Involvement:** The fever indicates that the infection has moved to other parts of the body (bacteremia) or is causing inflammation.

Clinical Implications:

- Severe fever and chills are indicators of a potentially life-threatening infection that may necessitate hospitalization.

- A persistent fever may be a sign of sepsis, a potentially fatal illness, particularly if it is accompanied by other symptoms like exhaustion or disorientation.

5.2 Excruciating flank or back pain

Another common sign of kidney infections is pain in the flanks or back. Inflammation of the renal tissue and adjacent tissues is usually the cause of this pain.

Features of Flank or Back Pain:

Location and Nature of Pain:

- Usually, pain is felt right below the ribs on one or both sides of the lower back.

- Depending on the degree of inflammation, it may spread to the groin or abdomen.

- Sharp, throbbing, or persistent pain are common descriptions of the condition.

Exacerbation with Movement:

- The discomfort may worsen with physical activity or even simple movements like twisting or bending.

Reasons for Pain in Kidney Infections

Kidney Inflammation:

- Pyelonephritis makes the kidneys swell, which creates pain signals by stretching the renal capsule.

Obstruction in the Urinary Tract:

- By raising the pressure inside the kidney, diseases such kidney stones or blockages can make the discomfort worse.

Referred Pain:

- Pain radiating to the flank or back may be caused by irritation of the diaphragm or adjacent muscles.

Clinical Considerations:

- In order to rule out complications such an abscess or blockage, severe or persistent discomfort requires prompt medical attention.
- Analgesics and antibiotic medication may be necessary for pain control in order to treat the infection.

5.3 General malaise, nausea, and vomiting

Upper UTIs frequently cause systemic symptoms such nausea, vomiting, and a strong feeling of being sick (malaise). The body's attempt to fend against a serious infection is frequently reflected in these symptoms.

Vomiting and Nausea
Characteristics:

- Patients may have intermittent or chronic nausea.
- Vomiting can happen suddenly or after meals, increasing the risk of dehydration.

Mechanisms:

- The kidneys contribute to electrolyte balance maintenance. Unbalances can lead to gastrointestinal irritation when they become inflamed.

- Toxins released by bacteria have the ability to activate the vagus nerve, which can result in nausea and vomiting.

General Malaise

Weakness and Fatigue:

- Systemic inflammation can result in excessive fatigue and the incapacity to carry out daily tasks.

- Patients may experience weakness, dizziness, or fatigue.

Loss of Appetite:

- Nausea and a general sense of being ill are major causes of disinterest in eating.

Mental Fog or Confusion:

- In extreme situations, particularly in elderly individuals, malaise may manifest as cognitive symptoms such as disorientation or trouble focusing.

Clinical Implications:

- Dehydration brought on by persistent nausea and vomiting may necessitate intravenous fluids.
- Loss of appetite and malaise point to the need for close observation, supportive treatment, and rest.

Upper urinary tract infections differ significantly from lower urinary tract infections in that they are characterized by unique and frequently severe symptoms. Signs of kidney involvement include high fever, chills, severe flank or back pain, and systemic symptoms including malaise and nausea. Since untreated upper urinary tract infections can result in potentially fatal consequences like sepsis or kidney damage, these symptoms emphasize the urgency of seeking medical attention. Early detection of these symptoms and appropriate care can guarantee a speedy recovery and avoid long-term effects.

CHAPTER 6

SYMPTOMS OF UTIS IN PARTICULAR GROUPS

Because of age, physiological changes, and medical conditions, urinary tract infections (UTIs) present differently in different groups. Because symptoms can be subtle, unusual, or linked to particular hazards, certain populations such as children, pregnant women, and older adults need to be more vigilant. This chapter offers a thorough examination of UTI symptoms in various populations, including information on how they manifest, their underlying causes, and the significance of prompt diagnosis.

6.1 Children's Symptoms: Parental Warning Signs

Children's UTIs are frequent and frequently difficult to diagnose because their symptoms might mimic those of other pediatric illnesses. In order to spot early symptoms and seek medical help, parents and other caregivers are essential.

Typical Children's Symptoms

Infants and Toddlers:

Fever:

- Fever is frequently the only symptom in young children.

- Prolonged weeping or fussiness, particularly when urinating, is a sign of irritability.

- A decrease in appetite or trouble nursing are signs of poor feeding.

- **Diarrhea and Vomiting:** General gastrointestinal problems.

- **Foul-smelling or cloudy urine:** Notable alterations when changing diapers.

Painful Urination (Dysuria):

Older Children:

- Complaints of a burning feeling when urinating.

- **Increased Urgency or Frequency**: recurrent bathroom visits with minimal results.

- **Back or Abdominal Pain:** Localized ache in the flanks or lower abdomen.

- **Bedwetting:** New episodes of bedwetting in

children who were previously potty trained.

Difficulties in Diagnosing UTIs in Children:

- **Non-Specific Symptoms:** A lot of symptoms might be mistaken for other conditions, like gastroenteritis or teething problems.

- **Communication Barriers:** Younger kids could find it difficult to express their distress.

- **Risk of Kidney Involvement:** Children's UTIs have a higher chance of moving up to the kidneys, where they can cause pyelonephritis if left untreated.

The Value of Parental Watchfulness

- Keep an eye out for any changes in urine habits or an inexplicable fever.

- Seek medical attention as soon as possible since children who have untreated UTIs may develop kidney damage.

6.2 Pregnancy-Related Risks and Symptoms

Because of hormonal changes and the mechanical pressure from the expanding uterus, pregnant women are more likely to get UTIs. In order to avoid difficulties for both mother and child, it is crucial to identify and treat UTIs in this population.

Pregnant women often experience pain, urgency, and frequent urination. These symptoms are similar to those of non-pregnant adults.

There may also be lower abdomen pain and urine that is hazy or smells bad.

Distinct Signs and Side Effects:

- **Raised Risk of Pyelonephritis**: High temperature, chills, and flank pain are possible symptoms.
- **Contractions or Cramping:** The signs of premature labor can occasionally be mistaken for UTIs.

Reasons for Increased Susceptibility During Pregnancy:

Hormonal Changes:

- Progesterone slows urine flow and increases the risk of bacterial development by relaxing the muscles of the urinary tract.
- The expanding uterus may compress the bladder, causing partial emptying. This is known as

mechanical compression.

Weakened Immune Response:

- The immune system changes throughout pregnancy, making the body less capable of fending against diseases.

Dangers of Pregnancy-Related UTIs:

- Preterm Labor: If left untreated, UTIs may result in early contractions and delivery.

- **Low Birth Weight:** Linked to kidney-infecting illnesses.

- **Preeclampsia:** This condition of elevated blood pressure may be exacerbated by severe illnesses.

The Value of Prompt Treatment:

- In order to prevent infections, routine prenatal care involves screening for asymptomatic bacteriuria, or bacteria in the urine without symptoms.

- Women who are pregnant should notify their healthcare physician right once if they experience any odd urine symptoms.

6.3 Older Adult Symptoms: Perplexity and Unusual Presentations

The diagnosis of UTIs can be difficult in older persons because they frequently have unusual or nonspecific symptoms. These variations are a result of both physiological and cognitive changes that occur with aging.

Typical Atypical Symptoms in Older Adults

Delirium or Confusion:

- Abrupt shifts in mental state, such as agitation, amnesia, or disorientation, could be the initial indication of a urinary tract infection.
- It's frequently confused with the onset of dementia or other neurological conditions.

Generalized Weakness:

- A discernible drop in vitality or heightened exhaustion.

Falls:

- UTIs can increase the risk of falls by impairing coordination or causing dizziness.

Appetite Loss:

- A decrease in food desire or inexplicable weight

loss.

Why Older Adult Symptoms Vary

Blunted Immune reaction:

- As people age, their bodies' inflammatory reaction is diminished, which leads to a decrease in common symptoms like fever or dysuria.

Pre Existing Conditions:

- Long-term conditions like diabetes or neurological problems might obscure or make symptoms more difficult to perceive.
- The use of catheters for an extended period of time raises the incidence of UTIs and can lead to unusual symptoms.

The Value of Early Identification

Risk of Complications:

- In older persons, particularly those with compromised immune systems, UTIs can rapidly escalate to sepsis.

Caregiver Awareness:

- Family members and caregivers should check for sudden behavioral changes or indicators of discomfort.

Because of their distinct symptomatology and related hazards, UTIs in specific populations—children, pregnant women, and older adults—need to be treated with caution. Non-specific symptoms in children, such as fever and agitation, necessitate parental attention. Women who are pregnant are more vulnerable and need to be aware of the hazards to their health as well as the health of the fetus. A high index of suspicion must be maintained by caregivers and healthcare professionals since older persons frequently exhibit bewilderment or generalized weakness. In order to ensure timely and efficient treatment, reduce problems, and encourage recovery in these susceptible populations, it is imperative to recognize these variances.

<h1 style="text-align:center">CHAPTER 7</h1>

<h2 style="text-align:center">UNTREATED UTI COMPLICATIONS</h2>

Urinary tract infections (UTIs) can develop into serious, occasionally fatal illnesses if left untreated. Even while many UTIs may be successfully treated with prompt action, neglecting to treat them can lead to problems that impact the kidneys, urinary system, and even the body as a whole. This chapter highlights the significance of early detection and treatment by examining the main consequences linked to untreated UTIs.

7.1 Development of Sepsis or Kidney Infections

Untreated UTIs have the potential to spread from the bladder and urethra in the lower urinary tract to the kidneys and ureters in the upper urinary system. Serious side effects like sepsis and renal infections may arise from this progression.

Pyelonephritis (Kidney Infections)

Mechanism of Progression:

- Bacteria can move from the bladder to the kidneys via the ureters, causing kidney tissue irritation and infection.

- The classic indications of pyelonephritis include a high temperature, chills, excruciating back or flank pain, nausea, and vomiting.

- If the infection is not treated, it may lead to abscesses or worsen renal function.

The Life-Threatening Complication of Sepsis

- The definition and mechanism of sepsis are as follows: The body's reaction to an infection results in extensive inflammation, which can induce organ malfunction and even failure.

- Urosepsis (sepsis originating in the urinary system) is frequently caused by UTIs, especially those that climb to the kidneys.

- Sepsis symptoms include a fast heartbeat, low blood pressure, disorientation, trouble breathing, and severe weakness.

- A life-threatening consequence of progressing to septic shock is multi-organ failure.

The Value of Early Intervention:

- Sepsis and kidney infections are medical emergencies that need to be treated right away. Hospitalization, intravenous antibiotics, and supportive care are all part of the treatment.

7.2 Chronic UTIs: An Understanding of Recurrent Infections

Recurrent UTIs, defined as three or more infections within a year or two within six months, constitute a substantial issue for individuals and healthcare providers.

Reasons for Recurrent UTIs
Incomplete Treatment:

- Bacteria in the urinary system may result from inadequate antibiotic therapy or patient noncompliance.

- The growth of biofilms on the bladder wall or urinary catheters can protect germs against antibiotics, making them persistent reservoirs of bacteria.

Underlying Conditions:

- Recurrent infections may be caused by kidney stones, structural problems, or neurogenic bladder dysfunction.

Changes in Women After Menopause:

- Lower estrogen levels might alter the microbiomes in the vagina and urine, making a person more vulnerable.

Repercussions of Prolonged UTIs

Impact on Quality of Life:

- Recurrent infections may result in frequent medical visits, chronic pain, and urgency in the urine.
- Regular use of antibiotics may encourage the emergence of resistant bacterial strains, making treatment more difficult in the future.

Management Techniques

Preventive Measures:

- Changing behavior, including drinking more water and maintaining good hygiene, might lessen recurrence.

Prophylactic Antibiotics:

- People who experience recurrences frequently may be offered low-dose antibiotics.

Treatment of Underlying Conditions:

- Long-term management requires addressing structural abnormalities or other contributing factors.

7.3 Urinary Tract Long-Term Damage

Severe or persistent UTIs can harm the urinary system irreparably, affecting its functionality and having long-term health effects.

Bladder Damage

Decreased Bladder Capacity:

- The bladder's capacity to efficiently store urine may be diminished by recurring inflammation and scarring.

Chronic Pain Syndromes:

- Recurrent infections can lead to the development of conditions such as interstitial cystitis (painful bladder syndrome).

Kidney Damage

Renal Scarring:

- Chronic kidney infections can reduce kidney function and raise the risk of chronic kidney disease (CKD) by causing scarring.

Hypertension:

- Scarring-induced renal impairment can raise blood pressure, which increases the risk of cardiovascular disease.

Elevated Risk of Subsequent Complications

Stone Formation:

- Urinary tract infections can encourage the development of urinary stones, which can worsen infections and further impede urine flow.

Urinary Incontinence:

- Loss of control over one's urine may result from damage to the bladder or sphincter processes.

The consequences of untreated UTIs highlight how important prompt diagnosis and treatment are. Recurrent infections and long-term urinary tract damage can seriously lower quality of life, while kidney infections or sepsis can have potentially fatal outcomes. The main tactics for reducing these consequences are prevention, efficient treatment, and addressing underlying risk factors. Patients and healthcare professionals can collaborate to avoid the severe consequences of untreated UTIs by being aware of the possible hazards.

CHAPTER 8

UTI Diagnosis

For a urinary tract infection (UTI) to be effectively treated and consequences to be avoided, an accurate and prompt diagnosis is crucial. Clinical assessment, laboratory tests, and, if necessary, sophisticated diagnostic methods are all used in the diagnosis process. The diagnostic procedure for UTIs is covered in detail in this chapter, along with the instruments and methods that medical professionals employ to verify the existence of infection and assess its severity.

8.1 Clinical Signs: What Physicians See

A comprehensive evaluation of clinical symptoms is the first stage in the diagnosis of a UTI. To direct additional testing, doctors depend on visible indicators and patient-reported experiences.

Important Signs of a UTI

Less common UTIs (Cystitis):

- Dysuria, or painful urination, frequent desires to urinate, and discomfort in the pelvic or bladder region.

Upper UTIs (Pyelonephritis):

- Signs of kidney involvement include chills, nausea, vomiting, high fever, and excruciating back pain.

Atypical Presentations:

- Fever, irritability, or poor eating are possible signs in youngsters.
- Rather than the usual symptoms, older persons frequently show signs of perplexity or general malaise.

The Significance of Medical History

Recurrent UTIs:

- Doctors evaluate the frequency and trends of previous infections to estimate the probability of recurrence.

Risk factors:

- Menopause, recent sex, spermicide use, and catheter use could all be contributing factors.

- Individuals who have diabetes, kidney stones, or structural abnormalities of the urinary tract may be at risk for UTIs.

Physical Examination

Abdominal and Back Assessment:

- Lower abdominal or flank tenderness indicates kidney or bladder involvement.
- Fever, dehydration, or exhaustion are examples of general health indicators that could point to a systemic infection.

8.2 Laboratory Tests: An Overview of Urinalysis and Urine Culture

Laboratory testing is essential for verifying the diagnosis and determining the causal organism following clinical assessment.

Urinalysis: The Initial Examination

What It Identifies:

- **White blood cells, or leukocytes:** Their presence indicates infection or inflammation.

- **Nitrites:** A bacterial infection is characterized by the conversion of urine nitrates to nitrites by bacteria like Escherichia coli.

- **Hematuria:** Blood in the urine could be a sign of urinary tract irritation or infection.

- **Proteinuria:** In severe situations, an excess of protein may indicate kidney damage.

Collection Method:

- To reduce contamination, a clean-catch midstream urine sample is usually utilized.

- Patients who are unable to deliver a clean sample may require catheterized samples.

Quick Results:

- Urinalysis offers prompt information, frequently accessible in a matter of minutes, assisting in the prompt formulation of treatment plans.

Finding the Causative Organism in Urine Culture

Goal:

- To identify the particular pathogen and verify the existence of a bacterial infection.

- The procedure involves incubating the urine sample to promote the growth of microorganisms.

- To assess the severity of an infection, colony-forming units (CFUs) are counted; >100,000 CFU/mL indicates a serious infection.

By examining patterns of bacterial resistance, antibiotic sensitivity testing determines which antibiotics are best for a given situation.

Laboratory Test Limitations

False Positives/Negatives:

- Low bacterial numbers or contaminated samples may result in incorrect diagnoses.

Cultural Time Delay:

- Specific treatments may be delayed as results take 24 to 72 hours. In the interval, empirical therapy is frequently started.

8.3 Complex Cases: Advanced Diagnostic Methods

Advanced diagnostic methods are used when routine tests are equivocal or when UTIs are complicated or recurrent.

Imaging Studies:

Goal:

- To assess any structural anomalies, blockages, or issues such kidney stones or abscesses.

One of the most used modalities is ultrasound, which is safe and non-invasive for identifying anatomical problems like stones or hydronephrosis.

- The CT scan offers detailed imaging that can be used to identify structural abnormalities, abscesses, or serious infections.
- When radiation exposure is a problem or in complex circumstances, MRI is utilized.

Cystoscopy

Procedure:

- To view the bladder and urethra directly, a thin, flexible tube equipped with a camera is placed into the urethra.

When It's Used:

- For anatomical anomalies, suspected malignancies, or recurring UTIs.
- One benefit is that it offers a clear view of the

urinary tract for diagnosis and, if necessary, biopsy.

Voiding Cystourethrogram (VCUG):

Goal:

- Assesses vesicoureteral reflux (VUR), a disorder in which urine empties into the kidneys from the bladder.

Who Needs It:

- Usually carried out on kids who have congenital defects or recurrent UTIs.

Specific Laboratory Examinations

Polymerase Chain Reaction (PCR):

- Allows for the quick and accurate diagnosis of diseases by detecting bacterial DNA in urine.

Blood Tests:

- Used to detect systemic illness (e.g., increased white blood cell count, inflammatory markers) and evaluate kidney function (e.g., creatinine, BUN).

When to Speak with an Expert

Urologist Referral:

- Suggested for complicated or recurring conditions

that call for sophisticated imaging or surgery.

Referral to Nephrologist:

Required when serious infections impair kidney function.

A mix of clinical expertise and laboratory accuracy is needed to diagnose a UTI. Urinalysis and urine culture offer conclusive proof, whereas clinical signs direct early suspicion. In complicated or recurring diseases, advanced diagnostic techniques like imaging and cystoscopy are quite helpful. A methodical approach guarantees precise diagnosis, directs focused therapy, and reduces the possibility of problems.

CHAPTER 9

UTI TREATMENT: SYMPTOM RELIEF

Eliminating the infection, reducing symptoms, and avoiding recurrence are the main goals of effective treatment for urinary tract infections (UTIs). Although antibiotics continue to be the mainstay of treatment, supportive care and symptom management are essential for a full recovery. This chapter looks at the main methods of treating UTIs, including at-home treatments and medical procedures, and offers advice on how to deal with discomfort while recovering.

9.1 Antibiotic Therapy: Options and Things to Think About

The main treatment for bacterial UTIs is antibiotics. Effective treatment while lowering the risk of resistance depends on the choice, dosage, and length of therapy.

Antibiotics that are frequently prescribed:

For Uncomplicated UTIs (Lower UTIs):

- **Trimethoprim-sulfamethoxazole (TMP-SMX):** A first-line option for many UTIs because of its efficacy against E. coli.

- With little effect on gut flora, nitrofurantoin is an effective treatment for bladder infections.

- **Fosfomycin:** A one-time treatment for germs that are resistant.

For Kidney Infections or Complicated UTIs:

- Fluoroquinolones (e.g., Ciprofloxacin, Levofloxacin): Beneficial for more severe or higher urinary tract infections, but used sparingly because of resistance issues.

- Pregnant women and people with medication sensitivities are frequently prescribed cephalosporins.

- **Carbapenems:** Saved for infections that are resistant to multiple drugs.

Antibiotic Use Considerations:

- **Tailoring to the Pathogen:** Urine culture results

inform antibiotic selection, guaranteeing focused therapy.

- For simple situations, the therapy will last three to five days.
- 7–14 days for pyelonephritis or complex UTIs.
- The following patient-specific factors need to be taken into account: age, renal function, pregnant status, and history of antibiotic allergies.

Antibiotic Resistance Issues

Emerging Resistance Patterns:

- Treatment has become more difficult due to resistant bacterial strains caused by overuse or misuse of antibiotics.

Combating Resistance:

- Completing prescribed courses and avoiding needless antibiotic use are crucial measures.

9.2 DIY Solutions: Drinking Water and Cranberry Juice

Home remedies can aid in the body's healing process and relieve mild symptoms while drugs treat the underlying issue.

Maintaining Hydration

Value of Fluids:

- Consuming enough water lowers the bacterial burden by flushing bacteria out of the urinary system.

- Regular urination also avoids urine stagnation, which can encourage the growth of pathogens.

It is advised that you consume eight to ten glasses of water per day.

- Steer clear of sugary or caffeinated drinks as they can irritate the bladder.

The Function of Cranberry Juice

Mechanism of Action:

- Proanthocyanidins, which are found in cranberries, are substances that stop bacteria, especially E. coli, from sticking to the lining of the urinary system.

- Research indicates that cranberry products may lower the risk of recurring UTIs, especially in women. They cannot, however, be used in place of antibiotics.

Usage Advice:

- To stay away from additional sugars, choose unsweetened cranberry juice or supplements.

- Consult a medical professional to be sure it will work with current therapies.

Additional Helpful Steps

Warm Compresses:

- The discomfort brought on by bladder spasms can be eased by placing a warm pad on the lower abdomen.

- **Dietary Adjustments:** Steer clear of alcohol, artificial sweeteners, and spicy meals to lessen bladder discomfort.

- **Supplements:** Probiotics, particularly strains such as Lactobacillus, help keep the gut and urinary microbiota in a healthy balance, which may lessen the likelihood of recurrent UTIs.

9.3 Handling Symptoms During the Healing Process

Improving comfort and quality of life throughout rehabilitation requires symptom alleviation.

Pain Management Over-the-Counter

Nonsteroidal Anti-Inflammatory Drugs (NSAIDs):

- Ibuprofen and other medications lower inflammation, which relieves fever and pain.

- Analgesic for the urinary tract that momentarily reduces burning and urgency feelings is phenazopyridine. Note: It can result in strong orange urine coloring and only cures the symptoms, not the infection itself.

Lifestyle Modifications for Comfort

Rest and Recovery:

- It's critical to avoid physically demanding activities during recovery in order to give the body time to mend.

- Frequent urination is important. Holding pee can worsen symptoms and lengthen the infection.

Clothing Options:

- Wearing breathable, loose materials, such as cotton underwear, lessens irritation and keeps moisture from accumulating.

Tracking Progress

Timeline for Symptom Resolution:

- After beginning antibiotics, symptoms often go away 48–72 hours later. If symptoms are persistent or getting worse, you should see a doctor right away.

Warning Signs of Complications:

- Urgent care is necessary if you have a high temperature, excruciating back pain, or sepsis symptoms (such as a fast heartbeat or confusion).

Targeted antibiotic therapy, supportive home remedies, and symptom management techniques are all used in the treatment of UTIs. Patients can find relief and lower their risk of consequences by treating the infection and any related discomfort. Antibiotics are still the mainstay of treatment, but lifestyle modifications and symptom monitoring are crucial to healing.

CHAPTER 10

LIFESTYLE AND HYGIENE ADVICE FOR PREVENTING UTIs

It is crucial to prevent urinary tract infections (UTIs), particularly in those who are prone to recurring infections. The incidence of UTIs can be considerably decreased by following good cleanliness habits, altering one's diet, and knowing when to consult a doctor. This chapter explores these tactics and offers practical advice for preserving urinary health and averting infections in the future.

10.1 Personal Hygiene Best Practices

Preventing the entry of bacteria into the urinary tract is mostly dependent on practicing good personal hygiene. Particularly in high-risk individuals, simple yet effective habits can reduce the risk of UTIs.

Women's Hygiene Advice

Wiping Front to Back:

- To avoid bacteria moving from the anus to the urethra, always wipe from the front to the back after using the restroom.

Urinating After Sexual Activity:

- Bacteria can enter the urethra as a result of sexual activity. Urinating soon after sexual activity aids in the removal of these microorganisms.

Avoid Harsh Products:

- Avoid douches, scented feminine hygiene sprays, and perfumed soaps since they might upset the vaginal flora's natural equilibrium and make you more prone to infections.

Overall Personal Hygiene for Every Gender

- **Regular Handwashing:** To stop the spread of bacteria, wash your hands well both before and after using the restroom.

- **Adequate Genital Care:** Use a mild soap and water to clean the genital area every day. Men who are not circumcised should carefully pull back their foreskin to clean below.

- **Changing Underwear Frequently:** To minimize bacterial growth, choose cotton or other breathable, moisture-wicking materials and stay away from tight-fitting underwear.

Extra Things to Think About

- **Avoid Prolonged Moisture Exposure**: To stop bacteria from growing, quickly change out of sweaty sports attire or wet swimsuits.
- **Conscientious Product Use:** To reduce the risk of infection, avoid using urinary catheters for extended periods of time and make sure they are properly sterilized.

10.2 Modifications to Diet to Promote Urinary Health

Dietary decisions can have a significant impact on preserving urinary tract health and lowering the risk of infections.

Maintaining Hydration:

- **Importance of Water:** Drinking lots of water helps dilute urine, which reduces the amount of space available for germs to thrive. Additionally, it encourages frequent urine, which eliminates bacteria.

- **Hydration Guidelines:** Try to drink 8 to 10 glasses of water per day, or more if you live in a hot area or exercise vigorously.

Nutrients and Foods That Help

Cranberries, which are high in proanthocyanidins, help to keep germs like E. coli from sticking to the lining of the urinary system. Choose supplements or unsweetened cranberry juice.

Probiotics:

- Foods that promote a healthy balance of gut and urinary microbiota, such as yogurt, kefir, and fermented vegetables, can help prevent infections.

- Citrus fruits, strawberries, and supplements raise the acidity of urine, which inhibits the growth of bacteria. This is the effect of vitamin C.

Foods to Steer Clear of:

- **Irritants:** Steer clear of coffee, alcohol, spicy foods, and artificial sweeteners since these might aggravate the symptoms of a urinary tract infection.

- **Sugary Foods:** Too much sugar can encourage the

growth of bacteria, raising the risk of infection.

Other Nutritional Techniques

- **Incorporate Fiber:** A diet high in fiber promotes regular bowel movements, which lowers the risk of constipation, which may indirectly lead to urinary tract infections.

- **Take a Look at Herbal Teas:** Because of their moderate diuretic qualities, teas like dandelion, green tea, or nettle may promote kidney and bladder health.

10.3 When to Get Expert Assistance for Repeated UTIs

Many UTIs can be avoided with lifestyle and hygiene changes, but recurring or persistent infections may need medical attention and treatment.

Identifying Recurrent UTIs

- **Recurrent UTI Definition:** A UTI is deemed recurrent if it occurs twice in a six-month period or three times in a year.

- **Common Signs:** Recurring infection episodes or

symptoms that don't go away even after therapy.

When to Speak with a Medical Professional

- **Persistent Symptoms:** See a doctor if UTI symptoms don't go away a few days after beginning medication.

- Severe symptoms, such as a high fever, excruciating flank or back pain, or indications of a systemic infection, necessitate prompt medical attention.

- **Underlying Medical Conditions:** Individuals who have kidney stones, diabetes, or urinary tract anatomical anomalies should get evaluated as soon as possible.

Diagnostic and Proactive Measures

- **Sophisticated Diagnostic Tests:** Imaging tests or cystoscopy might be suggested to detect structural irregularities or issues.

- A low-dose antibiotic regimen may be recommended for people who have recurrent UTIs in order to prevent further infections.

- **Immunoprophylaxis:** Vaccines that target bacteria that cause UTIs are examples of emerging therapeutics.

A proactive strategy that incorporates good cleanliness, wise food choices, and prompt medical attention for recurring instances is needed to prevent UTIs. By taking these precautions, the incidence of infections can be considerably decreased, and general urinary health can be improved. Knowing when to seek expert help guarantees timely care, reduces problems, and preserves long-term health.

ABOUT THE AUTHOR

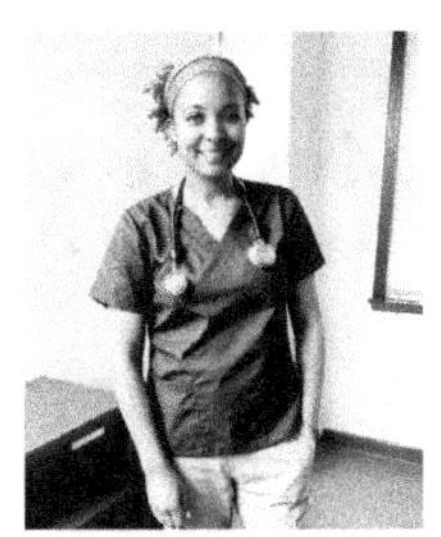

Harmony Royce is a dedicated healthcare worker who has a strong interest in holistic wellness. Harmony's extensive history in various aspects of health and wellness provides her with a wealth of knowledge and expertise that she can utilize in her writing and professional endeavors.

Harmony is a talented author who crafts thought-provoking books that inspire readers to have well-rounded, balanced lives. She writes about a variety of health-related topics, such as diet, exercise, mental health, and mindfulness. Her approachable writing style combines practical guidance with evidence-based research to make complex health concepts approachable and engaging for readers of all ages.

Harmony actively promotes the benefits of holistic health through writing, community workshops, and internet forums. Her mission is to educate and inspire people about the transformative power of self-care and healthy lifestyle choices.